Mediterranean Diet

for

Osteoporosis

"Embark on a transformative journey through the Mediterranean's culinary wisdom for optimal bone health

JAMIE KIM

TABLE OF CONTENTS

INTRODUCTION

Understanding Osteoporosis

Understanding Osteoporosis involves grasping the key aspects of this bone-related condition

What is Osteoporosis?

Osteoporosis is a medical condition where bones become brittle and fragile, leading to an increased risk of fractures. This happens because the density and quality of the bone are reduced.

Causes and Risk Factors:

Age:

Osteoporosis is more common in older adults as bone density naturally decreases with age.

Gender:

Women, especially after menopause, are at a higher risk due to hormonal changes affecting bone density.

Family History:

If a family member has osteoporosis, it may increase your risk.

Low Body Weight:

People with a small body frame or low body weight may have less bone mass.

Hormonal Changes:

Hormonal imbalances, such as low estrogen or testosterone, can contribute.

How Osteoporosis Develops:

Bone Remodeling:

Bones are in a constant state of renewal, with old bone being replaced by new. In osteoporosis, this balance is disrupted.

Bone Density Loss:

Gradually, more bone is lost than formed, leading to a decrease in bone density.

Symptoms:

Silent Disease:

Osteoporosis is often called a "silent disease" as it progresses without noticeable symptoms until a fracture occurs.

Common Fracture Sites:

Fractures commonly occur in the hip, spine, and wrist.

Prevention and Management:

Healthy Lifestyle:

Adequate calcium and vitamin D intake through diet or supplements.

Regular Exercise:

Weight-bearing exercises help maintain bone density.

Avoiding Smoking and Excessive Alcohol:

Both can contribute to bone loss.

Bone Density Tests:

Regular screenings to assess bone health.

Conclusion:

Understanding osteoporosis involves recognizing its risk factors, how it develops, and the importance of preventive measures. By adopting a bone-healthy lifestyle, individuals can take proactive steps to reduce the risk of osteoporosis and enhance overall bone health.

Importance of Diet in Managing Osteoporosis

Calcium and Vitamin D Intake:

Calcium: Essential for bone strength. A diet rich in dairy products, leafy greens, and fortified foods helps meet calcium needs.

Vitamin D: Facilitates calcium absorption. Sun exposure, fatty fish, and fortified foods contribute to vitamin D intake.

Protein for Bone Structure:

Proteins provide the building blocks for bone structure. Include lean meats, poultry, fish, dairy, beans, and nuts in your diet.

Magnesium and Phosphorus Balance:

Magnesium and phosphorus work alongside calcium for bone health. Incorporate whole grains, nuts, seeds, and green vegetables into your meals.

Vitamin K for Bone Mineralization:

Vitamin K supports bone mineralization. Green leafy vegetables, broccoli, and certain oils are good sources.

Antioxidants and Anti-Inflammatory Foods:

Fruits and vegetables rich in antioxidants help reduce inflammation, promoting overall bone health.

Limiting Sodium and Caffeine:

Excessive sodium and caffeine can lead to calcium loss. Moderation in consumption supports bone density.

Balancing Acidic and Alkaline Foods:

Diets high in acidic foods (meat, processed foods) may impact calcium balance. Balancing with alkaline foods (fruits, vegetables) is beneficial.

Maintaining a Healthy Weight:

A balanced diet helps manage weight, reducing stress on bones. Obesity and underweight both pose risks to bone health.

Hydration:

Staying adequately hydrated is essential for bone health. Water supports overall bodily functions, including those related to bone metabolism.

Omega-3 Fatty Acids:

Found in fatty fish, flaxseeds, and walnuts, omega-3 fatty acids have anti-inflammatory properties beneficial for bone health.

Customizing Diet to Individual Needs:

Tailoring the diet to personal preferences and any existing health conditions ensures a sustainable approach to managing osteoporosis.

Overview of the Mediterranean Diet

The Mediterranean Diet is more than just a culinary choice; it's a lifestyle that emphasizes the traditional dietary patterns of countries bordering the Mediterranean Sea. Renowned for its health benefits, this diet is characterized by an abundance of fresh, whole foods and a focus on heart-healthy fats. Here's a comprehensive overview:

Foundation of Fresh Produce:

Fruits and Vegetables: The diet centers around a variety of colorful fruits and vegetables, rich in vitamins, minerals, and antioxidants.

Whole Grains and Legumes:

- **Whole Grains:** Emphasis on whole grains like barley, quinoa, and whole wheat for sustained energy.
- **Legumes:** Beans, lentils, and chickpeas provide a source of protein and fiber.

Healthy Fats:

- **Olive Oil:** The primary source of fat, known for its monounsaturated fats and anti-inflammatory properties.

- **Nuts and Seeds:** Almonds, walnuts, and flaxseeds contribute to heart-healthy fats.

Lean Proteins:

- **Fish and Seafood:** Regular consumption of fatty fish like salmon and mackerel for omega-3 fatty acids.
- **Poultry:** Limited intake of lean poultry like chicken and turkey.
- **Dairy:** Moderate consumption of Greek yogurt and cheese for calcium.

Moderate Wine Consumption:

Red Wine: In moderation, typically with meals, providing antioxidants and heart-protective compounds.

Herbs and Spices:

- **Fresh Herbs:** Basil, oregano, and rosemary add flavor without the need for excess salt.
- **Spices:** Mediterranean cuisines use spices like garlic and cumin for taste and potential health benefits.

Limited Red Meat:

Occasional Red Meat: Red meat, especially lean cuts, is consumed in moderation.

Social and Physical Activity:

- **Regular Physical Activity:** The diet is complemented by an active lifestyle, promoting overall well-being.
- **Social Engagement:** Shared meals with family and friends are a cornerstone of the Mediterranean lifestyle.

Emphasis on Seasonal and Local Foods:

Fresh and Seasonal: Utilizing locally sourced, seasonal ingredients for optimal freshness and sustainability.

Adaptability and Customization:

Flexibility: The Mediterranean Diet is adaptable, allowing for cultural and personal variations while maintaining its core principles.

Health Benefits:

- **Heart Health:** Linked to reduced risk of heart disease and stroke.
- **Weight Management:** Supports healthy weight maintenance.
- **Anti-Inflammatory Effects:** Rich in foods with anti-inflammatory properties.

In essence, the Mediterranean Diet offers a holistic approach to nutrition, emphasizing whole foods, a balance of macronutrients, and a lifestyle that extends beyond what's on the plate. Its proven health benefits make it a compelling choice for those seeking a sustainable and enjoyable way to support overall well-being.

CHAPTER ONE

FOUNDATIONS OF THE MEDITERRANEAN DIET

Key Principles

The Mediterranean Diet is characterized by a set of fundamental principles that form the basis of its nutritional philosophy. Understanding and incorporating these key principles can help individuals derive maximum health benefits from this dietary approach:

Plant-Based Focus:

The majority of meals should center around a variety of fresh fruits, vegetables, whole grains, legumes, nuts, and seeds.

Heart-Healthy Fats:

Prioritize monounsaturated fats, predominantly found in olive oil, as the primary source of dietary fat. Additionally, include moderate amounts of nuts and seeds for added healthy fats.

Lean Proteins:

Emphasize lean protein sources, such as fish and seafood, which are rich in omega-3 fatty acids. Poultry, eggs, and dairy products are consumed in moderation, while red meat is limited.

Whole Grains:

Choose whole grains like brown rice, quinoa, and whole wheat over refined grains, promoting sustained energy and greater nutritional content.

Moderate Wine Consumption:

If alcohol is consumed, do so in moderation, with an emphasis on red wine during meals, owing to its potential cardiovascular benefits.

Herbs and Spices Instead of Salt:

Flavor meals with fresh herbs, garlic, and a variety of spices instead of excessive salt. This enhances taste while reducing sodium intake.

Regular Physical Activity:

Integrate regular physical activity into daily life, aligning with the Mediterranean lifestyle's emphasis on holistic well-being.

Social Connections:

Foster a sense of community and social engagement, often achieved through shared meals with family and friends.

Seasonal and Locally Sourced Foods:

Prioritize fresh, seasonal, and locally sourced ingredients, supporting both environmental sustainability and optimal nutritional content.

Customization and Flexibility:

Adapt the diet to individual preferences, cultural influences, and health needs while maintaining the core principles.

Mindful Eating:

Cultivate mindful eating habits, savoring and appreciating the flavors of each meal. Pay attention to hunger and fullness cues.

Variety and Balance:

Aim for a diverse and balanced diet, incorporating a range of food groups to ensure a broad spectrum of nutrients.

Water as the Primary Beverage:

Hydrate with water as the primary beverage, limiting the consumption of sugary drinks and excessive caffeine.

Food Groups and Portions

Understanding the appropriate food groups and portions is essential for adopting and benefiting from the Mediterranean Diet. Here's a breakdown of the key components and recommended proportions:

Fruits and Vegetables:

Recommendation: Make fruits and vegetables the foundation of your meals.

Portion: Aim for at least 5 servings of fruits and vegetables per day, emphasizing a colorful variety.

Whole Grains:

Recommendation: Choose whole grains for their fiber and nutrient content.

Portion: Make whole grains a staple, aiming for 3 to 4 servings daily. Examples include whole wheat, barley, quinoa, and brown rice.

Lean Proteins:

Recommendation: Prioritize fish and seafood, legumes, and lean poultry.

Portion: Include fish in meals at least twice a week. Moderate portions of poultry, legumes, and eggs are also encouraged.

Healthy Fats:

Recommendation: Use olive oil as the primary source of fat.

Portion: Incorporate 2 to 4 tablespoons of olive oil daily, whether in cooking or as a dressing for salads.

Nuts and Seeds:

Recommendation: Include a variety of nuts and seeds for added nutrients.

Portion: Consume a small handful (about 1 ounce) of nuts or seeds several times a week.

Dairy Products:

Recommendation: Choose low-fat or fat-free dairy options, such as Greek yogurt and cheese.

Portion: Limit dairy consumption to moderate portions, incorporating it into meals and snacks.

Moderate Wine Consumption:

Recommendation: If you drink alcohol, do so in moderation.

Portion: For wine, moderation typically means up to one glass per day for women and up to two glasses per day for men, preferably with meals.

Herbs and Spices:

Recommendation: Use herbs and spices generously for flavoring instead of excessive salt.

Portion: Experiment with a variety of herbs and spices, adjusting to personal taste preferences.

Water:

- **Recommendation:** Stay hydrated with water as the primary beverage.
- **Portion:** Drink at least 8 glasses (64 ounces) of water daily, adjusting based on individual needs and physical activity.

Sweets and Desserts:

Recommendation: Limit intake of sweets and desserts, focusing on natural sweetness from fruits.

Portion: Enjoy desserts occasionally and in small portions.

Coffee and Tea:

Recommendation: Moderate consumption of coffee and tea is acceptable.

Portion: Limit caffeine intake to moderate levels, considering individual tolerance.

Customization:

Recommendation: Tailor portions based on individual energy needs, activity levels, and health goals.

Portion: Listen to your body's hunger and fullness cues to guide your portion sizes.

Benefits of the Mediterranean Diet for Bone Health

The Mediterranean Diet, known for its numerous health advantages, offers specific benefits that contribute to the overall well-being of bones. Here's how adopting this dietary pattern can positively impact bone health:

Rich in Calcium and Vitamin D:

The diet includes calcium-rich foods such as dairy products, leafy greens, and fortified foods, ensuring an adequate intake for bone strength.

Sunlight exposure, a component of the Mediterranean lifestyle, contributes to natural vitamin D synthesis.

Optimal Nutrient Balance:

A variety of fruits, vegetables, whole grains, and lean proteins provide a well-balanced mix of nutrients necessary for bone health, including magnesium, phosphorus, and vitamin K.

Anti-Inflammatory Properties:

The Mediterranean Diet, abundant in fruits, vegetables, and olive oil, possesses anti-inflammatory properties that may help reduce inflammation, which is associated with bone loss.

Omega-3 Fatty Acids:

Fatty fish, a staple in the diet, is a rich source of omega-3 fatty acids. These essential fats contribute to bone health and may reduce the risk of osteoporosis.

Moderate Protein Intake:

The diet includes moderate amounts of lean proteins, supporting muscle health and overall bone density.

Weight Management:

The Mediterranean Diet, coupled with an active lifestyle, helps maintain a healthy weight. Excess body weight can strain bones, and weight management is crucial for preventing bone-related issues.

Reduced Sodium Intake:

The diet emphasizes the use of herbs and spices for flavoring instead of excessive salt. Lower sodium intake contributes to better calcium retention in the bones.

Whole Foods for Bone Density:

Whole grains, a key component of the diet, provide essential nutrients for bone density, including magnesium and phosphorus.

Balanced Acid-Alkaline Ratio:

The diet's emphasis on a variety of fruits and vegetables helps maintain a balanced acid-alkaline ratio in the body, which is associated with better bone health.

Hydration:

Adequate water consumption is encouraged, supporting overall health and hydration, which is vital for maintaining the flexibility of bones.

Lifestyle Factors:

Regular physical activity, another integral part of the Mediterranean lifestyle, promotes bone health by enhancing bone density and strength.

Customizable for Individual Needs:

The flexibility of the Mediterranean Diet allows individuals to customize it to meet their unique dietary preferences and needs while still promoting bone health.

CHAPTER TWO

NUTRIENT-RICH FOODS FOR BONE STRENGTH

Calcium-Rich Choices

1. Milk

2. Yogurt

3. Cheese (especially hard cheeses like cheddar)

4. Fortified plant-based milk (soy, almond, oat)

5. Fortified orange juice

6. Tofu (with added calcium sulfate)

7. Edamame

8. Collard greens

9. Kale

10. Broccoli

11. Bok choy

12. Okra

13. Almonds

14. Sesame seeds

15. Chia seeds

16. Canned sardines (with bones)

17. Canned salmon (with bones)

18. Canned shrimp

19. Fortified cereals

20. Fortified tofu

21. Spinach

22. Turnip greens

23. Mustard greens

24. Cabbage

25. Figs (dried)

26. Oranges

27. Kiwi

28. Papaya

29. Fortified plant-based yogurt

30. Fortified plant-based cheese

31. Molasses

32. White beans

33. Navy beans

34. Black-eyed peas

35. Chickpeas

36. Lentils

37. Fortified rice milk

38. Fortified coconut milk

39. Fortified almond milk

40. Fortified hemp milk

41. Fortified cashew milk

42. Fortified breakfast bars

43. Fortified waffles

44. Fortified instant oatmeal

45. Fortified rice cereal

46. Fortified whole grain bread

47. Fortified tortillas

48. Fortified pasta

49. Fortified dried fruits (apricots, raisins)

50. Fortified energy bars

Vitamin D Sources

1. Fatty fish (salmon, mackerel, trout, tuna)

2. Cod liver oil

3. Sardines

4. Fortified cow's milk

5. Fortified plant-based milk (soy, almond, oat)

6. Fortified orange juice

7. Fortified yogurt

8. Fortified cereal

9. Egg yolks

10. Beef liver

11. Cheese (especially Swiss and cheddar)

12. Fortified margarine

13. Mushrooms (exposed to sunlight)

14. Fortified tofu

15. Fortified soy milk

16. Fortified rice milk

17. Fortified almond milk

18. Fortified coconut milk

19. Fortified cereals

20. Fortified energy bars

21. Herring

22. Caviar

23. Shrimp

24. Oysters

25. Anchovies

26. Swordfish

27. Maitake mushrooms

28. Shiitake mushrooms

29. UV-exposed wild-caught fish

30. UV-exposed farmed fish

31. Halibut

32. Rainbow trout

33. Fortified butter

34. Fortified cheese spreads

35. Pork ribs

36. Goat cheese

37. Emmental cheese

38. Gruyère cheese

39. Bluefin tuna

40. Mackerel

41. Eel

42. Catfish

43. Swordfish

44. Whitefish

45. Tilapia

46. Egg whites (small amounts)

47. Fortified chocolate milk

48. Fortified plant-based cheese

49. Fortified plant-based yogurt

50. Fortified plant-based spreads (margarine

Magnesium and Phosphorus in the Diet

Both magnesium and phosphorus are essential minerals that play vital roles in various physiological functions within the body. Understanding their sources and significance in the diet is crucial for maintaining overall health.

Magnesium

Food Sources:

- Leafy green vegetables (spinach, kale)
- Nuts and seeds (almonds, pumpkin seeds)
- Whole grains (brown rice, quinoa, whole wheat)

- Legumes (black beans, chickpeas)
- Fish (mackerel, salmon)
- Avocado
- Bananas
- Dark chocolate

Functions:

- Supports bone health by aiding calcium absorption.
- Facilitates muscle function and relaxation.
- Contributes to energy production.
- Regulates blood pressure.
- Plays a role in over 300 enzymatic reactions in the body.

Recommended Daily Intake:

- Adult males: 400-420 mg
- Adult females: 310-320 mg

Phosphorus

Food Sources:

- Dairy products (milk, cheese, yogurt)
- Meat and poultry (beef, chicken, turkey)
- Fish (salmon, tuna)
- Eggs

- Nuts and seeds (sunflower seeds, pumpkin seeds)
- Whole grains (whole wheat, brown rice)
- Legumes (lentils, chickpeas)

Functions:

- Integral to the formation and maintenance of bones and teeth.
- Essential for energy metabolism.
- Involved in DNA and RNA synthesis.
- Acts as a buffer to maintain acid-base balance in the body.

Recommended Daily Intake:

- Adult males and females: 700 mg

Balancing Magnesium and Phosphorus

- While both minerals are crucial, an appropriate balance is necessary. An excessive intake of phosphorus, often found in processed foods and sodas, can impact magnesium absorption.
- A diet rich in whole foods, including fruits, vegetables, nuts, seeds, and whole grains, can contribute to a balanced intake of magnesium and phosphorus.

Considerations:

Individuals with certain medical conditions or those taking medications may need to monitor their magnesium and phosphorus levels closely.

Always consult with a healthcare professional or a registered dietitian for personalized dietary recommendations.

CHAPTER THREE

MEDITERRANEAN DIET AND WEIGHT MANAGEMENT

Maintaining a Healthy Weight

Achieving and sustaining a healthy weight is vital for overall well-being and the prevention of various health issues. Here are key principles and practices for maintaining a healthy weight:

Balanced Diet:

- Consume a well-balanced diet that includes a variety of fruits, vegetables, whole grains, lean proteins, and healthy fats.
- Pay attention to portion sizes to avoid overeating, and be mindful of calorie intake.

Regular Physical Activity:

- Engage in regular physical activity to burn calories and improve overall fitness.
- Aim for at least 150 minutes of moderate-intensity exercise or 75 minutes of vigorous-intensity exercise per week.

Strength Training:

Include strength training exercises to build and maintain lean muscle mass, which can boost metabolism and aid in weight management.

Hydration:

Stay adequately hydrated by drinking water throughout the day. Sometimes, the body can misinterpret thirst as hunger, leading to unnecessary calorie consumption.

Mindful Eating:

Eat slowly and savor each bite. Being mindful of the eating process can help prevent overeating and promote a healthier relationship with food.

Healthy Snacking:

Choose nutrient-dense snacks such as fruits, vegetables, nuts, or yogurt to curb hunger between meals.

Limit Processed Foods and Sugars:

- Reduce the intake of processed foods, sugary beverages, and snacks high in added sugars.
- Opt for whole, unprocessed foods to provide essential nutrients without excessive calories.

Regular Meal Times:

Establish regular meal times to regulate appetite and prevent mindless eating throughout the day.

Adequate Sleep:

Ensure sufficient and quality sleep, as lack of sleep can disrupt hormonal balance and contribute to weight gain.

Stress Management:

Manage stress through techniques like meditation, deep breathing, or regular physical activity. Chronic stress can lead to emotional eating and weight gain.

Accountability:

Keep a food diary or use apps to track meals, snacks, and physical activity. This can raise awareness and aid in making healthier choices.

Set Realistic Goals:

Establish realistic and achievable weight-related goals. Small, gradual changes are more sustainable than drastic measures.

Impact on Bone Density

Bone density refers to the amount of bone tissue in a certain volume of bone. It is a critical aspect of bone health and is influenced by various factors. Here are some key points regarding the impact on bone density:

Nutrition:

- Adequate intake of calcium and vitamin D is crucial for maintaining optimal bone density. These nutrients are essential for the formation and mineralization of bone tissue.
- A diet lacking in calcium and vitamin D can lead to reduced bone density, making bones more susceptible to fractures and osteoporosis.

Physical Activity:

- Weight-bearing exercises, such as walking, running, and weightlifting, stimulate bone remodeling and help maintain or increase bone density.
- Sedentary lifestyles or lack of physical activity can contribute to lower bone density over time.

Hormonal Factors:

- Hormones play a significant role in bone health. Estrogen, in particular, is important for maintaining bone density in women. Postmenopausal women may experience a decline in estrogen levels, leading to a reduction in bone density and an increased risk of osteoporosis.

- In men, low levels of testosterone can also contribute to decreased bone density.

Age:

- Bone density tends to peak in early adulthood, and after that, there is a gradual decline. This is a natural part of the aging process.

- As people age, the rate of bone resorption (breakdown) may exceed the rate of bone formation, resulting in decreased bone density.

Medical Conditions and Medications:

- Certain medical conditions, such as rheumatoid arthritis, celiac disease, and hormonal disorders, can affect bone density.

- Some medications, including glucocorticoids and certain anticonvulsants, may also contribute to bone loss.

Genetics:

- Genetic factors influence bone density and can contribute to an individual's susceptibility to conditions like osteoporosis.

- Family history of fractures or osteoporosis may indicate a genetic predisposition to lower bone density.

Lifestyle Choices:

Smoking and excessive alcohol consumption have been linked to lower bone density. Both habits can interfere with the body's ability to absorb calcium and can negatively impact bone health.

Maintaining healthy bone density is important for overall skeletal health and can help prevent fractures and bone-related conditions. Adopting a balanced diet, engaging in regular physical activity, avoiding harmful habits, and managing underlying health conditions are key components of maintaining optimal bone density throughout life

CHAPTER FOUR

INCORPORATING ANTI-INFLAMMATORY FOODS

Role of Inflammation in Osteoporosis

Inflammation plays a complex and multifaceted role in the development and progression of osteoporosis, a condition characterized by weakened bones and an increased risk of fractures.

Bone Resorption and Inflammatory Cytokines:

- Inflammation can stimulate the production of certain pro-inflammatory cytokines, such as interleukin-1 (IL-1), interleukin-6 (IL-6), and tumor necrosis factor-alpha (TNF-α).

- These cytokines can enhance the activity of osteoclasts, cells responsible for bone resorption. An increased rate of bone resorption without proper bone formation can lead to a net loss of bone density.

Chronic Inflammatory Conditions:

- Chronic inflammatory conditions, such as rheumatoid arthritis, systemic lupus erythematosus, and inflammatory bowel diseases, are associated with an increased risk of osteoporosis.

- In these conditions, the chronic activation of the immune system and elevated levels of inflammatory markers contribute to accelerated bone loss.

Glucocorticoid-Induced Osteoporosis:

- Long-term use of glucocorticoid medications, commonly prescribed for conditions like rheumatoid arthritis and asthma, is a significant risk factor for osteoporosis.

- Glucocorticoids can induce bone loss by promoting osteoclast activity, inhibiting osteoblast function (cells responsible for bone formation), and causing apoptosis (programmed cell death) of osteoblasts.

Osteoimmunology:

- Osteoimmunology is an interdisciplinary field that explores the interactions between the skeletal and immune systems. Inflammation is a central component of these interactions.

- Immune cells, such as T cells and macrophages, participate in bone remodeling processes.

Dysregulation of these interactions, often seen in inflammatory conditions, can lead to imbalances in bone turnover.

Estrogen and Inflammation:

- Estrogen has anti-inflammatory effects, and its decline, such as during menopause, can contribute to increased inflammation.
- Postmenopausal women, who experience a decrease in estrogen levels, are at an elevated risk of osteoporosis due in part to the pro-inflammatory environment that may accelerate bone loss.

Therapeutic Implications:

- Targeting inflammation is an area of interest in osteoporosis management. Medications that suppress inflammation, such as anti-resorptive agents like bisphosphonates or denosumab, may be prescribed to reduce bone turnover and prevent further bone loss.
- However, the use of these medications should be carefully considered, taking into account the individual's overall health and the specific underlying causes of inflammation.

In summary, inflammation contributes to osteoporosis by promoting bone resorption, disrupting the balance of bone remodeling, and influencing the function of bone cells. Understanding the interplay between inflammation and bone health is crucial for developing effective strategies to prevent and manage osteoporosis, especially in individuals with chronic inflammatory conditions or those undergoing long-term glucocorticoid therapy.

Mediterranean Foods with Anti-Inflammatory Properties

The Mediterranean diet is renowned for its potential health benefits, including its anti-inflammatory properties. This eating pattern is rich in fruits, vegetables, whole grains, nuts, seeds, and olive oil, while also incorporating moderate amounts of fish, poultry, and dairy. Here are some Mediterranean foods known for their anti-inflammatory properties.

Olive Oil:

Extra virgin olive oil is a staple in the Mediterranean diet and is rich in monounsaturated fats and antioxidants, such as polyphenols. These components have been shown to have anti-inflammatory effects.

Fruits and Vegetables:

- Berries (e.g., blueberries, strawberries)
- Leafy greens (e.g., spinach, kale)
- Tomatoes
- Broccoli
- Bell peppers
- Garlic
- Onions

These foods are packed with vitamins, minerals, fiber, and various phytonutrients that possess anti-inflammatory properties.

Fatty Fish:

- Salmon
- Mackerel
- Sardines
- Anchovies

Fatty fish are high in omega-3 fatty acids, particularly EPA (eicosapentaenoic acid) and DHA (docosahexaenoic acid), which have anti-inflammatory effects.

Nuts and Seeds:

- Almonds
- Walnuts

- Flaxseeds
- Chia seeds

These are good sources of healthy fats, fiber, and antioxidants, contributing to the anti-inflammatory nature of the Mediterranean diet.

Whole Grains:

- Whole wheat
- Brown rice
- Quinoa
- Barley

Whole grains provide fiber and a range of nutrients that can help reduce inflammation.

Legumes:

- Chickpeas
- Lentils
- Black beans

Legumes are rich in fiber, protein, and various anti-inflammatory compounds.

Herbs and Spices:

- Turmeric
- Ginger

- Rosemary
- Thyme
- Basil

These herbs and spices contain bioactive compounds with anti-inflammatory properties.

Yogurt and Cheese:

- Greek yogurt
- Feta cheese

These dairy products provide probiotics (beneficial bacteria) and calcium, which can contribute to a healthy inflammatory response.

Red Wine (in moderation):

Red wine, when consumed in moderation, contains resveratrol, a polyphenol with potential anti-inflammatory effects.

Avocado:

Avocados are rich in monounsaturated fats, which have been associated with anti-inflammatory effects. They also contain various vitamins, minerals, and antioxidants.

Citrus Fruits:

- Oranges

- Grapefruits
- Lemons

Citrus fruits are high in vitamin C, which is a powerful antioxidant with anti-inflammatory properties.

Pomegranate:

Pomegranates contain polyphenols and antioxidants, including punicalagins and anthocyanins, which contribute to their anti-inflammatory effects.

Herbal Teas:

- Chamomile tea
- Peppermint tea
- Green tea

Herbal teas, especially those with anti-inflammatory herbs like chamomile and mint, can be soothing and contribute to overall health.

Eggs:

Eggs, particularly those rich in omega-3 fatty acids, can be part of a Mediterranean-style diet. They provide essential nutrients and proteins.

Dark Chocolate (in moderation):

Dark chocolate with a high cocoa content contains flavonoids, which have antioxidant and anti-inflammatory properties. Moderation is key due to its calorie and sugar content.

Tahini:

Tahini, made from sesame seeds, is a source of healthy fats, vitamins, and minerals. It can be used in dressings, dips, and spreads.

Mushrooms:

Mushrooms, especially varieties like shiitake and maitake, contain bioactive compounds that may have anti-inflammatory effects.

Cinnamon:

Cinnamon has anti-inflammatory and antioxidant properties and can be added to various dishes, including oatmeal and yogurt.

Whole Grain Pasta:

Whole grain pasta provides fiber and nutrients, offering a healthier alternative to refined pasta.

Seaweed:

Seaweed, commonly consumed in Mediterranean countries, is rich in minerals, vitamins, and antioxidants that may contribute to anti-inflammatory effects.

47

CHAPTER FIVE

MEAL PLANNING AND RECIPES

1000 Days Recipes

1. Mediterranean Salmon Salad:

Ingredients:

- 2 salmon fillets
- Mixed salad greens
- Cherry tomatoes, halved
- Cucumber, sliced
- Kalamata olives
- Feta cheese, crumbled
- Olive oil and lemon dressing

Instructions:

- Season salmon with olive oil, lemon juice, salt, and pepper. Bake until cooked.
- Toss salad greens, tomatoes, cucumber, olives, and feta.
- Top the salad with the cooked salmon.
- Drizzle with olive oil and lemon dressing.

Nutritional Value (per serving):

- Protein: ~25g

- Calcium: ~150mg

- Vitamin D: ~10mcg

- Omega-3 fatty acids

Serving Methods:

- Serve as a main course for lunch or dinner.

- Prepare smaller portions for a nutrient-packed salad bowl.

2. Quinoa Stuffed Bell Peppers:

Ingredients:

- Bell peppers, halved

- Quinoa, cooked

- Chickpeas, drained

- Spinach, chopped

- Feta cheese, crumbled

- Garlic, minced

- Olive oil

Instructions:

- Mix cooked quinoa, chickpeas, spinach, feta, and garlic.

- Stuff bell peppers with the quinoa mixture.

- Drizzle with olive oil and bake until peppers are tender.

Nutritional Value (per serving):

- Protein: ~15g

- Calcium: ~100mg

- Fiber: ~8g

- Iron: ~3mg

Serving Methods:

- Serve as a vegetarian main dish.

- Pair with grilled chicken or fish for added protein.

3. Mediterranean Chickpea Salad:

Ingredients:

- Chickpeas, cooked

- Cherry tomatoes, halved

- Cucumber, diced

- Red onion, finely chopped

- Feta cheese, crumbled

- Kalamata olives

- Fresh parsley, chopped

- Olive oil and balsamic vinegar dressing

Instructions:

- Combine chickpeas, tomatoes, cucumber, red onion, feta, olives, and parsley.

- Toss with olive oil and balsamic vinegar dressing.
- **Nutritional Value (per serving):**
- Protein: ~12g
- Fiber: ~8g
- Calcium: ~100mg
- Vitamin C: ~30mg

Serving Methods:

- Serve as a refreshing side dish.
- Spoon over whole grain pita bread for a satisfying wrap.

4. Mediterranean Quiche with Spinach and Feta:

Ingredients:

- Whole wheat pie crust
- Eggs
- Spinach, chopped
- Feta cheese, crumbled
- Cherry tomatoes, halved
- Red bell pepper, diced
- Milk or alternative (e.g., almond milk)

Instructions:

- Whisk eggs and milk together.
- Mix in spinach, feta, tomatoes, and bell pepper.

- Pour mixture into the pie crust and bake until set.
- **Nutritional Value (per serving):**
- Protein: ~15g
- Calcium: ~200mg
- Vitamin A: ~500 IU
- Vitamin K: ~50mcg

Serving Methods:

- Enjoy for a weekend brunch.
- Serve with a side salad for a complete meal.

5. Mediterranean Lentil Soup:

Ingredients:

- Lentils, rinsed
- Carrots, diced
- Celery, diced
- Onion, chopped
- Garlic, minced
- Tomatoes, diced
- Vegetable broth
- Olive oil
- Fresh lemon juice

Instructions:

- Sauté onions, garlic, carrots, and celery in olive oil.

- Add lentils, tomatoes, and vegetable broth. Simmer until lentils are cooked.

- Season with salt, pepper, and a squeeze of fresh lemon juice.

Nutritional Value (per serving):

- Protein: ~18g

- Fiber: ~10g

- Folate: ~200mcg

- Iron: ~4mg

Serving Methods:

- Serve as a hearty soup for lunch or dinner.

- Pair with whole grain bread for a complete meal.

6. Mediterranean Stuffed Zucchini:

Ingredients:

- Zucchini, halved

- Ground turkey or lean ground chicken

- Quinoa, cooked

- Cherry tomatoes, diced

- Red onion, finely chopped

- Feta cheese, crumbled

- Fresh mint, chopped

- Olive oil

Instructions:

- Hollow out zucchini halves.
- Sauté ground meat, tomatoes, and onion until cooked.
- Mix in cooked quinoa, feta, and mint.
- Stuff zucchini with the mixture and bake until zucchini is tender.

Nutritional Value (per serving):

- Protein: ~20g
- Fiber: ~5g
- Calcium: ~120mg
- Vitamin B6: ~0.5mg

Serving Methods:

- Serve as a wholesome dinner entree.
- Pair with a side of Greek yogurt or tzatziki.

7. Mediterranean Roasted Veggie and Chickpea Bowl:

Ingredients:

- Chickpeas, drained
- Eggplant, diced
- Zucchini, sliced

- Red bell pepper, chopped
- Red onion, sliced
- Cherry tomatoes, halved
- Olive oil and lemon dressing

Instructions:

- Toss chickpeas and vegetables in olive oil.
- Roast until vegetables are golden.
- Drizzle with olive oil and lemon dressing.

Nutritional Value (per serving):

- Protein: ~12g
- Fiber: ~10g
- Vitamin C: ~40mg
- Magnesium: ~80mg

Serving Methods:

- Enjoy as a satisfying lunch bowl.
- Serve over whole grain couscous or quinoa.

8. Greek-Style Spinach and Feta Stuffed Chicken Breast:

Ingredients:

- Chicken breasts, boneless and skinless
- Spinach, wilted and chopped

- Feta cheese, crumbled

- Sundried tomatoes, chopped

- Garlic, minced

- Lemon juice

Instructions:

- Mix spinach, feta, tomatoes, garlic, and lemon juice.

- Cut a pocket in each chicken breast and stuff with the mixture.

- Bake until chicken is cooked through.

Nutritional Value (per serving):

- Protein: ~30g

- Calcium: ~150mg

- Vitamin A: ~300 IU

- Vitamin C: ~10mg

Serving Methods:

- Serve as an elegant dinner dish.

- Pair with a side of quinoa or a Greek salad.

9. Mediterranean Shrimp and Vegetable Skewers:

Ingredients:

- Shrimp, peeled and deveined

- Cherry tomatoes

- Bell peppers, cut into chunks

- Red onion, cut into wedges

- Zucchini, sliced

- Olive oil and oregano marinade

Instructions:

- Marinate shrimp and vegetables in olive oil and oregano.

- Thread onto skewers and grill until shrimp is cooked.

- Serve with a squeeze of lemon.

Nutritional Value (per serving):

- Protein: ~25g

- Vitamin C: ~30mg

- Selenium: ~40mcg

- Zinc: ~2mg

Serving Methods:

- Enjoy as a light and flavorful dinner.

- Serve over a bed of quinoa or brown rice.

10. Mediterranean Lentil and Vegetable Wrap:

Ingredients:

- Whole grain wraps

- Lentils, cooked

- Hummus

- Cherry tomatoes, sliced

- Cucumber, julienned

- Red onion, thinly sliced

- Fresh parsley, chopped

Instructions:

- Spread hummus on each wrap.

- Layer with lentils, tomatoes, cucumber, onion, and parsley.

- Wrap and enjoy.

Nutritional Value (per serving):

- Protein: ~15g

- Fiber: ~10g

- Iron: ~3mg

- Vitamin K: ~50mcg

Serving Methods:

- Pack as a nutritious lunch option.

- Serve with a side of Greek yogurt or a simple salad.

11. Mediterranean Grilled Chicken Salad:

Ingredients:

- Chicken breasts, grilled and sliced
- Mixed salad greens
- Cherry tomatoes, halved
- Cucumber, sliced
- Red bell pepper, diced
- Kalamata olives
- Feta cheese, crumbled
- Olive oil and balsamic vinegar dressing

Instructions:

- Arrange salad greens on a plate.
- Top with grilled chicken, tomatoes, cucumber, bell pepper, olives, and feta.
- Drizzle with olive oil and balsamic vinegar dressing.

Nutritional Value (per serving):

- Protein: ~25g
- Vitamin A: ~400 IU
- Vitamin C: ~40mg
- Fiber: ~5g

Serving Methods:

- Serve as a light and satisfying lunch or dinner.

- Add a sprinkle of chopped fresh herbs, such as oregano or basil.

12. Mediterranean Eggplant and Tomato Bake:

Ingredients:

- Eggplant, sliced
- Tomatoes, sliced
- Red onion, thinly sliced
- Garlic, minced
- Olive oil
- Fresh basil, chopped
- Parmesan cheese, grated

Instructions:

- Layer eggplant, tomatoes, and onion in a baking dish.
- Drizzle with olive oil and sprinkle garlic, basil, and Parmesan.
- Bake until vegetables are tender.

Nutritional Value (per serving):

- Fiber: ~7g
- Vitamin K: ~30mcg
- Folate: ~40mcg
- Calcium: ~100mg

Serving Methods:

- Serve as a flavorful side dish.
- Pair with whole grain couscous or quinoa for a complete meal.

13. Mediterranean Tuna and White Bean Salad:

Ingredients:

- Canned tuna, drained
- Cannellini beans, drained
- Red onion, finely chopped
- Cherry tomatoes, halved
- Fresh parsley, chopped
- Lemon juice
- Olive oil

Instructions:

- Combine tuna, beans, onion, tomatoes, and parsley.
- Dress with lemon juice and olive oil.
- Toss gently and chill before serving.

Nutritional Value (per serving):

- Protein: ~20g
- Fiber: ~8g

- Vitamin C: ~20mg

- Iron: ~2mg

Serving Methods:

- Enjoy as a light lunch or dinner.

- Serve on whole grain crackers or as a filling for a pita pocket.

14. Mediterranean Sweet Potato and Chickpea Bake:

Ingredients:

- Sweet potatoes, cubed

- Chickpeas, drained

- Red bell pepper, sliced

- Red onion, diced

- Garlic, minced

- Olive oil and cumin seasoning

Instructions:

- Toss sweet potatoes, chickpeas, bell pepper, and onion with olive oil and cumin.

- Roast until sweet potatoes are tender.

- Garnish with fresh herbs, like cilantro.

Nutritional Value (per serving):

- Protein: ~10g

- Fiber: ~8g

- Vitamin A: ~300 IU

- Vitamin C: ~30mg

Serving Methods:

- Serve as a vegetarian main course.

- Top with a dollop of Greek yogurt or tahini sauce.

15. Mediterranean Shrimp and Quinoa Bowl:

Ingredients:

- Shrimp, sautéed

- Quinoa, cooked

- Cherry tomatoes, halved

- Cucumber, diced

- Red onion, finely chopped

- Feta cheese, crumbled

- Olive oil and lemon dressing

Instructions:

- Arrange quinoa in bowls.

- Top with sautéed shrimp, tomatoes, cucumber, onion, and feta.

- Drizzle with olive oil and lemon dressing.

Nutritional Value (per serving):

- Protein: ~20g

- Fiber: ~5g

- Calcium: ~150mg

- Vitamin D: ~10mcg

Serving Methods:

- Serve as a well-balanced dinner bowl.

- Add a squeeze of fresh lemon juice for extra flavor.

16. Greek Lemon-Herb Baked Chicken:

Ingredients:

- Chicken thighs, bone-in and skin-on

- Lemon juice

- Olive oil

- Fresh oregano, chopped

- Garlic, minced

- Salt and pepper

Instructions:

- Marinate chicken in a mixture of lemon juice, olive oil, oregano, garlic, salt, and pepper.

- Bake until chicken is golden and cooked through.

Nutritional Value (per serving):

- Protein: ~25g

- Vitamin C: ~20mg

- Iron: ~2mg

- Vitamin B6: ~0.5mg

Serving Methods:

- Serve with a side of roasted vegetables.

- Pair with a quinoa or couscous salad.

17. Mediterranean Stuffed Portobello Mushrooms:

Ingredients:

- Portobello mushrooms, stems removed

- Quinoa, cooked

- Spinach, sautéed

- Sun-dried tomatoes, chopped

- Feta cheese, crumbled

- Balsamic glaze

Instructions:

- Fill mushrooms with a mixture of quinoa, sautéed spinach, sun-dried tomatoes, and feta.

- Bake until mushrooms are tender.

- Drizzle with balsamic glaze before serving.

Nutritional Value (per serving):

- Protein: ~12g

- Fiber: ~8g

- Calcium: ~100mg

- Vitamin D: ~5mcg

Serving Methods:

- Enjoy as a vegetarian main course.

- Serve alongside a green salad.

18. Mediterranean Cauliflower Rice Bowl:

Ingredients:

- Cauliflower rice, cooked

- Grilled chicken or chickpeas

- Cherry tomatoes, halved

- Cucumber, diced

- Olives, sliced

- Hummus

- Tzatziki sauce

Instructions:

- Arrange cauliflower rice in bowls.

- Top with grilled chicken or chickpeas, tomatoes, cucumber, and olives.

- Drizzle with hummus and tzatziki.

Nutritional Value (per serving):

- Protein: ~15g

- Fiber: ~10g

- Vitamin K: ~30mcg

- Iron: ~2mg

Serving Methods:

- Serve as a light and nourishing lunch.

- Customize with your favorite Mediterranean toppings.

19. Mediterranean Quinoa and Vegetable Stir-Fry:

Ingredients:

- Quinoa, cooked

- Mixed vegetables (bell peppers, zucchini, cherry tomatoes)

- Red onion, sliced

- Chickpeas, cooked

- Feta cheese, crumbled

- Lemon vinaigrette

Instructions:

- Stir-fry vegetables and chickpeas in a pan.

- Mix in cooked quinoa.

- Drizzle with lemon vinaigrette and top with feta.

Nutritional Value (per serving):

- Protein: ~10g
- Fiber: ~8g
- Vitamin C: ~40mg
- Calcium: ~100mg

Serving Methods:

- Serve as a quick and healthy weeknight dinner.
- Add a sprinkle of fresh herbs, such as parsley or basil.

20. Mediterranean Herb-Marinated Grilled Swordfish:

Ingredients:

- Swordfish steaks
- Fresh lemon juice
- Olive oil
- Garlic, minced
- Fresh herbs (rosemary, thyme, oregano), chopped
- Salt and pepper

Instructions:

- Marinate swordfish in a mixture of lemon juice, olive oil, garlic, herbs, salt, and pepper.
- Grill until fish is cooked through.

Nutritional Value (per serving):

- Protein: ~30g
- Vitamin D: ~15mcg
- Omega-3 fatty acids
- Selenium: ~50mcg

Serving Methods:

- Serve with a side of quinoa or couscous.
- Pair with a Mediterranean salsa made with tomatoes, olives, and capers.

21. Mediterranean Lentil and Vegetable Stew:

Ingredients:

- Green lentils, rinsed
- Carrots, diced
- Celery, chopped
- Onion, finely chopped
- Garlic, minced
- Crushed tomatoes
- Vegetable broth
- Olive oil
- Fresh parsley, chopped

Instructions:

- Sauté onions, garlic, carrots, and celery in olive oil.
- Add lentils, crushed tomatoes, and vegetable broth.
- Simmer until lentils are tender.
- Garnish with fresh parsley before serving.

Nutritional Value (per serving):

- Protein: ~15g
- Fiber: ~12g
- Vitamin A: ~500 IU
- Iron: ~3mg

Serving Methods:

- Serve as a comforting stew for lunch or dinner.
- Pair with whole grain bread or a side salad.

22. Greek-Style Quinoa and Chickpea Patties:

Ingredients:

- Quinoa, cooked
- Chickpeas, mashed
- Red onion, finely chopped
- Feta cheese, crumbled
- Fresh dill, chopped
- Lemon zest
- Whole grain flour

- Olive oil

Instructions:

- Mix quinoa, mashed chickpeas, onion, feta, dill, and lemon zest.
- Form patties, coat with flour, and pan-fry in olive oil.
- Serve with a yogurt-based tzatziki sauce.

Nutritional Value (per serving):

- Protein: ~12g
- Fiber: ~8g
- Calcium: ~150mg
- Vitamin C: ~10mg

Serving Methods:

- Serve as a delicious vegetarian main dish.
- Wrap in whole grain pita with veggies for a Mediterranean-style burger.

23. Mediterranean Baked Cod with Tomatoes and Olives:

Ingredients:

- Cod fillets
- Cherry tomatoes, halved

- Kalamata olives, sliced

- Red onion, thinly sliced

- Garlic, minced

- Olive oil

- Fresh basil, chopped

Instructions:

- Place cod fillets in a baking dish.

- Top with tomatoes, olives, onion, and garlic.

- Drizzle with olive oil and bake until fish is cooked.

- Garnish with fresh basil before serving.

Nutritional Value (per serving):

- Protein: ~25g

- Vitamin C: ~20mg

- Omega-3 fatty acids

- Iron: ~2mg

Serving Methods:

- Serve as a light and flavorful dinner.

- Pair with a side of quinoa or couscous.

24. Mediterranean Chickpea and Spinach Stuffed Peppers:

Ingredients:

- Bell peppers, halved
- Chickpeas, cooked
- Spinach, sautéed
- Red onion, finely chopped
- Feta cheese, crumbled
- Lemon juice
- Olive oil

Instructions:

- Mix chickpeas, sautéed spinach, onion, feta, and lemon juice.
- Stuff bell peppers with the mixture.
- Drizzle with olive oil and bake until peppers are tender.

Nutritional Value (per serving):

- Protein: ~15g
- Fiber: ~8g
- Vitamin A: ~300 IU
- Calcium: ~100mg

Serving Methods:

- Serve as a vegetarian main dish.
- Pair with a side of Greek salad for a complete meal.

25. Mediterranean Roasted Red Pepper and Walnut Dip:

Ingredients:

- Roasted red peppers (from a jar)
- Walnuts
- Garlic, minced
- Olive oil
- Lemon juice
- Cumin
- Greek yogurt

Instructions:

- Blend roasted red peppers, walnuts, garlic, olive oil, lemon juice, and cumin in a food processor.
- Mix in Greek yogurt for a creamy consistency.
- Serve as a dip with vegetable sticks or whole grain pita.

Nutritional Value (per serving):

- Protein: ~6g
- Fiber: ~3g
- Vitamin C: ~30mg
- Iron: ~1mg

Serving Methods:

- Serve as a flavorful dip for a party or gathering.
- Spread on whole grain crackers or use as a sandwich spread.

26. Mediterranean Quinoa Salad with Avocado and Chickpeas:

Ingredients:

- Quinoa, cooked
- Cherry tomatoes, halved
- Cucumber, diced
- Red bell pepper, chopped
- Chickpeas, drained and rinsed
- Avocado, diced
- Feta cheese, crumbled
- Kalamata olives, sliced
- Olive oil and balsamic vinaigrette

Instructions:

- Combine quinoa, tomatoes, cucumber, bell pepper, chickpeas, avocado, feta, and olives.
- Drizzle with olive oil and balsamic vinaigrette.
- Toss gently before serving.

Nutritional Value (per serving):

- Protein: ~12g

- Fiber: ~8g

- Vitamin C: ~30mg

- Healthy fats

Serving Methods:

- Enjoy as a refreshing and filling lunch.

- Serve as a side dish at picnics or barbecues.

27. Mediterranean Stuffed Acorn Squash:

Ingredients:

- Acorn squash, halved

- Ground lamb or turkey

- Quinoa, cooked

- Spinach, sautéed

- Red onion, finely chopped

- Pine nuts

- Cinnamon and cumin

- Olive oil

Instructions:

- Roast acorn squash halves.

- Sauté ground meat, mix with cooked quinoa, sautéed spinach, onion, pine nuts, and spices.

- Fill acorn squash halves with the mixture.

Nutritional Value (per serving):

- Protein: ~20g
- Fiber: ~10g
- Vitamin A: ~500 IU
- Iron: ~3mg

Serving Methods:

- Serve as a festive dinner dish.
- Pair with a side of Greek yogurt or tzatziki.

28. Mediterranean Chickpea and Artichoke Tagine:

Ingredients:

- Chickpeas, cooked
- Artichoke hearts, quartered
- Tomatoes, diced
- Red onion, chopped
- Garlic, minced
- Ras el Hanout spice blend
- Olive oil
- Fresh cilantro, chopped

Instructions:

- Sauté onion and garlic in olive oil.

- Add chickpeas, artichoke hearts, tomatoes, and spice blend.
- Simmer until flavors meld.
- Garnish with fresh cilantro.

Nutritional Value (per serving):

- Protein: ~10g
- Fiber: ~8g
- Vitamin C: ~20mg
- Iron: ~2mg

Serving Methods:

- Serve over couscous or quinoa.
- Garnish with a dollop of Greek yogurt.

29. Mediterranean Turkey and Eggplant Skewers:

Ingredients:

- Ground turkey
- Eggplant, cubed
- Red onion, sliced
- Cherry tomatoes
- Olive oil and lemon marinade
- Oregano and garlic powder

Instructions:

- Mix ground turkey with oregano and garlic powder.

- Form meatballs and alternate with eggplant, onion, and tomatoes on skewers.

- Grill until cooked.

- Drizzle with olive oil and lemon marinade.

Nutritional Value (per serving):

- Protein: ~20g

- Vitamin C: ~15mg

- Healthy fats

- Vitamin A: ~200 IU

Serving Methods:

- Serve as a protein-packed dinner.

- Pair with a side of quinoa or a Greek salad.

30. Mediterranean Cauliflower and Chickpea Curry:

Ingredients:

- Cauliflower, florets

- Chickpeas, cooked

- Coconut milk

- Tomatoes, diced

- Onion, finely chopped

- Garlic, minced

- Curry spices (turmeric, cumin, coriander)

- Fresh cilantro, chopped

Instructions:

- Sauté onion and garlic in a pan.
- Add cauliflower, chickpeas, tomatoes, coconut milk, and curry spices.
- Simmer until cauliflower is tender.
- Garnish with fresh cilantro before serving.

Nutritional Value (per serving):

- Protein: ~15g
- Fiber: ~10g
- Vitamin C: ~40mg
- Iron: ~3mg

Serving Methods:

- Serve over brown rice or quinoa.
- Garnish with a squeeze of fresh lemon juice.

Meal Plans

- **Day 1:**

Breakfast: Greek-Style Quinoa and Chickpea Patties

Lunch: Mediterranean Salmon Salad

Dinner: Mediterranean Quinoa Salad with Avocado and Chickpeas

- **Day 2:**

Breakfast: Mediterranean Lentil Soup

Lunch: Greek-Style Spinach and Feta Stuffed Chicken Breast

Dinner: Mediterranean Cauliflower and Chickpea Curry

- **Day 3:**

Breakfast: Mediterranean Quiche with Spinach and Feta

Lunch: Mediterranean Sweet Potato and Chickpea Bake

Dinner: Mediterranean Baked Cod with Tomatoes and Olives

- **Day 4:**

Breakfast: Mediterranean Chickpea and Artichoke Tagine

Lunch: Mediterranean Turkey and Eggplant Skewers

Dinner: Mediterranean Eggplant and Tomato Bake

- **Day 5:**

Breakfast: Mediterranean Stuffed Acorn Squash

Lunch: Mediterranean Herb-Marinated Grilled Swordfish

Dinner: Mediterranean Roasted Red Pepper and Walnut Dip (as an appetizer) + Greek Lemon-Herb Baked Chicken

- **Day 6:**

Breakfast: Mediterranean Stuffed Zucchini

Lunch: Mediterranean Quinoa and Vegetable Stir-Fry

Dinner: Mediterranean Tuna and White Bean Salad

- **Day 7:**

Breakfast: Mediterranean Tuna and White Bean Salad (yes, it's versatile!)

Lunch: Mediterranean Grilled Chicken Salad

Dinner: Mediterranean Lentil Soup

- **Day 8:**

Breakfast: Mediterranean Shrimp and Quinoa Bowl

Lunch: Mediterranean Stuffed Portobello Mushrooms

Dinner: Greek-Style Quinoa and Chickpea Patties

- **Day 9:**

Breakfast: Mediterranean Lentil and Vegetable Stew

Lunch: Mediterranean Cauliflower Rice Bowl

Dinner: Mediterranean Herb-Marinated Grilled Swordfish

- **Day 10:**

Breakfast: Mediterranean Quinoa Salad with Avocado and Chickpeas

Lunch: Mediterranean Tuna and White Bean Salad

Dinner: Mediterranean Sweet Potato and Chickpea Bake

- **Day 11:**

Breakfast: Mediterranean Stuffed Zucchini

Lunch: Mediterranean Shrimp and Vegetable Skewers

Dinner: Mediterranean Chickpea and Spinach Stuffed Peppers

- **Day 12:**

Breakfast: Mediterranean Chickpea and Artichoke Tagine

Lunch: Mediterranean Stuffed Acorn Squash

Dinner: Mediterranean Quiche with Spinach and Feta

- **Day 13:**

Breakfast: Mediterranean Roasted Red Pepper and Walnut Dip

Lunch: Mediterranean Lentil and Vegetable Stew

Dinner: Mediterranean Baked Cod with Tomatoes and Olives

- **Day 14:**

Breakfast: Mediterranean Tuna and White Bean Salad (yes, it's versatile!)

Lunch: Mediterranean Shrimp and Quinoa Bowl

Dinner: Mediterranean Stuffed Portobello Mushrooms

CHAPTER SIX

LIFESTYLE FACTORS FOR BONE HEALTH

Exercise and Physical Activity

Walking:

Steps:

- Wear comfortable athletic shoes.
- Start with a brisk walk, swinging your arms naturally.
- Maintain good posture, keeping your head up and shoulders back.
- Walk for at least 30 minutes, gradually increasing intensity over time.
- Cool down with a slower-paced walk.

Bodyweight Squats:

Steps:

- Stand with feet shoulder-width apart.
- Lower your body by bending your knees and pushing your hips back.
- Keep your chest up and back straight.
- Lower until your thighs are parallel to the ground.

- Push through your heels to return to the starting position.

Push-Ups:

Steps:

- Start in a plank position with hands slightly wider than shoulder-width apart.
- Lower your body by bending your elbows.
- Keep your body in a straight line.
- Push back up to the starting position.
- Modify by doing push-ups on your knees if needed.

Jumping Jacks:

Steps:

- Stand with feet together and arms at your sides.
- Jump while spreading your legs and raising your arms overhead.
- Jump again, bringing your legs back together and arms to your sides.
- Repeat in a continuous, fluid motion.

Plank:

Steps:

- Start in a push-up position with arms straight.
- Lower onto your forearms.
- Keep your body in a straight line from head to heels.
- Hold the position, engaging your core muscles.
- Gradually increase the duration over time.

Lunges:

Steps:

- Stand with feet together.
- Take a step forward with one foot, lowering your body until both knees are bent.
- The back knee should hover just above the ground.
- Push off the front foot to return to the starting position.
- Repeat on the other leg.

Bicycle Crunches:

Steps:

- Lie on your back with hands behind your head.
- Lift your legs and bend your knees.
- Bring one knee towards your chest while straightening the other leg.

- Rotate your torso, bringing the opposite elbow towards the bent knee.

- Repeat on the other side in a cycling motion.

Burpees:

Steps:

- Start in a standing position.

- Drop into a squat position and place your hands on the ground.

- Jump your feet back into a plank position.

- Perform a push-up.

- Jump your feet towards your hands and explosively jump up.

Dumbbell Bicep Curls:

Steps:

- Hold a dumbbell in each hand, arms fully extended at your sides.

- Keep your elbows close to your torso.

- Curl the weights upward, contracting your biceps.

- Lower the weights back down with control.

- Repeat for the desired number of repetitions.

Yoga Sun Salutation:

Steps:

- Start in Mountain Pose (Tadasana).

- Inhale and raise your arms overhead (Urdhva Hastasana).

- Exhale and fold forward into Forward Bend (Uttanasana).

- Inhale, lift your torso, and extend your spine (Halfway Lift).

- Exhale, step or jump back into Plank, then lower into Chaturanga.

- Inhale into Upward-Facing Dog (Urdhva Mukha Svanasana).

- Exhale into Downward-Facing Dog (Adho Mukha Svanasana).

- Inhale and step or jump to the front of your mat.

- Exhale into Forward Bend and return to Mountain Pose.

Remember to warm up before exercising and cool down afterward. Adjust the intensity and repetitions based on your fitness level and gradually progress as your strength and endurance improve.

Sunlight Exposure for Vitamin D

1. Sunlight and Vitamin D Synthesis:

- **UVB Radiation:** Sunlight contains ultraviolet B (UVB) radiation, which is essential for the skin to produce vitamin D.

- **Skin Reaction:** When the skin is exposed to UVB rays, a cholesterol derivative in the skin converts to previtamin D3.

- **Conversion to Vitamin D:** Previtamin D3 is then converted into active vitamin D (calcitriol) through a series of chemical reactions.

2. Factors Influencing Vitamin D Production:

- **Geographical Location:** The angle of the sun's rays varies by location, affecting the intensity of UVB radiation. People living at higher latitudes may have reduced vitamin D synthesis during certain seasons.

- **Time of Day:** Sun exposure is most effective for vitamin D synthesis when the sun is high in the sky, typically between 10 a.m. and 3 p.m.

- **Skin Tone:** Darker skin requires more prolonged sun exposure to produce the same amount of vitamin D as lighter skin, as melanin reduces UVB absorption.

3. Duration of Sun Exposure:

- **Short Exposure:** For fair-skinned individuals, approximately 10–30 minutes of sun exposure to the face, arms, and legs a few times per week during peak sunlight hours may be adequate.
- **Extended Exposure:** Those with darker skin or living in regions with reduced sunlight may require longer exposure.

4. Sunscreen and Clothing:

- **Sunscreen Use:** Sunscreen with a high sun protection factor (SPF) can significantly reduce UVB absorption. However, even with sunscreen, some vitamin D synthesis can occur.
- **Clothing Coverage:** Covered skin limits UVB exposure, so exposing larger areas of skin facilitates vitamin D production.

5. Vitamin D and Health:

- **Bone Health:** Vitamin D is crucial for calcium absorption, contributing to bone health.
- **Immune System:** Adequate vitamin D levels are associated with a well-functioning immune system.
- **Mood Regulation:** Some studies suggest a link between vitamin D levels and mood regulation.

6. Supplementation Consideration:

- **Dietary Sources:** While sunlight is a natural source, vitamin D can also be obtained from certain foods such as fatty fish, fortified dairy products, and supplements.
- **Supplementation:** In cases where sunlight exposure is limited, and dietary intake is insufficient, vitamin D supplements may be recommended, especially for at-risk populations.

7. Health Guidelines:

Individual Variability: Vitamin D needs vary among individuals, and factors like age, health status, and lifestyle influence requirements.

Stress Management and Sleep

Stress management and sleep are closely interconnected aspects of overall well-being. Effectively managing stress contributes significantly to improved sleep quality, and conversely, getting adequate and restful sleep helps in coping with stress. Here are strategies for stress management and promoting better sleep:

Stress Management:

Mindfulness Meditation:

- Engage in mindfulness meditation to focus on the present moment, reducing stress and promoting mental clarity.
- Practice deep breathing exercises to enhance relaxation and alleviate tension.

Regular Exercise:

- Incorporate regular physical activity into your routine, such as walking, jogging, or yoga.
- Exercise helps release endorphins, which act as natural mood lifters and stress relievers.

Time Management:

- Prioritize tasks and set realistic goals to avoid feeling overwhelmed.
- Break down larger tasks into smaller, more manageable steps.

Social Support:

- Maintain strong social connections with friends and family.
- Share concerns and feelings with trusted individuals, fostering a sense of support.

Healthy Lifestyle:

- Adopt a balanced and nutritious diet to support physical and mental well-being.
- Limit caffeine and sugar intake, as excessive consumption can contribute to heightened stress.

Learn to Say No:

- Set boundaries and avoid overcommitting to responsibilities.
- Recognize the importance of personal time and relaxation.

Positive Visualization:

- Visualize positive outcomes and focus on solutions rather than dwelling on problems.
- Use positive affirmations to reinforce a constructive mindset.

Time for Hobbies:

- Engage in activities you enjoy and that bring you a sense of fulfillment.
- Hobbies can serve as effective stress outlets and contribute to overall well-being.

Sleep Promotion:

Establish a Sleep Routine:

- Maintain a consistent sleep schedule by going to bed and waking up at the same time every day.
- Create a calming bedtime routine to signal to your body that it's time to wind down.

Create a Comfortable Sleep Environment:

- Ensure your bedroom is conducive to sleep by keeping it dark, quiet, and cool.
- Invest in a comfortable mattress and pillows for optimal support.

Limit Screen Time Before Bed:

- Reduce exposure to screens (phones, tablets, computers) at least an hour before bedtime.
- The blue light emitted from screens can interfere with the production of the sleep-inducing hormone melatonin.

Mindful Relaxation Techniques:

- Practice relaxation techniques before bedtime, such as gentle yoga or progressive muscle relaxation.
- Consider activities like reading a book or taking a warm bath to unwind.

Limit Stimulants:

- Avoid consuming stimulants like caffeine or nicotine close to bedtime.

- Be mindful of the timing of evening meals to prevent discomfort during sleep.

Manage Stress Before Bed:

- Engage in stress-reducing activities in the evening to promote relaxation.

- Practice mindfulness or deep breathing exercises to calm the mind.

Evaluate Sleep Environment:

- Address any environmental factors that may disrupt sleep, such as noise or uncomfortable bedding.

- Consider using blackout curtains to minimize external light.

Professional Help:

- If sleep problems persist, consider seeking guidance from a healthcare professional or sleep specialist.

- Conditions like insomnia may benefit from cognitive-behavioral therapy for insomnia (CBT-I).

CONCLUSION

In conclusion, "Mediterranean Diet for Osteoporosis" serves as a holistic guide, unraveling the intricate relationship between nutrition, lifestyle, and bone health. Through a meticulous exploration of the Mediterranean diet's rich tapestry, this book has illuminated the profound impact of food choices on the prevention and management of osteoporosis.

The Mediterranean diet, renowned for its heart-healthy attributes, emerges as a compelling ally in fortifying bones and mitigating the risk of osteoporosis. From the abundance of nutrient-dense fruits and vegetables to the inclusion of omega-3-rich fish and the wholesome embrace of olive oil, each dietary component is a testament to the diet's ability to nourish bones with a symphony of essential vitamins and minerals.

Beyond nutrition, the book delves into the Mediterranean lifestyle, weaving together the threads of physical activity, stress management, and the conviviality of shared meals. It underscores the pivotal role of sunlight exposure in fostering vitamin D synthesis, a crucial element in the bone health narrative.

As readers journey through these pages, they are empowered with practical insights and a repertoire of flavorful, osteoporosis-friendly recipes that seamlessly integrate into everyday life. The culinary exploration not only enriches palates but also stands as a testament to the delectable synergy between health-conscious choices and gastronomic delight.

In the intricate dance of science and tradition, the Mediterranean Diet for Osteoporosis emerges as a roadmap, guiding individuals towards a lifestyle that not only safeguards their bone health but also enhances their overall well-being. It is a call to embrace a way of living that transcends the boundaries of mere sustenance, encapsulating the profound philosophy that what we put on our plates resonates deeply within the very foundation of our skeletal health.

Ultimately, this book is an invitation – an invitation to savor the vibrant flavors of the Mediterranean, to revel in the joy of movement, to find solace in mindful living, and above all, to fortify the body from within. It is a celebration of the remarkable interplay between food, culture, and health, offering a transformative narrative that empowers individuals to craft their own stories of resilience and bone vitality. As the final chapter unfolds, the readers are not merely closing a book; they are opening a chapter in their lives where the wisdom of the Mediterranean diet becomes a cherished companion on the journey to lasting bone health and a life well-lived.

99